CW00519330

A BEGINNER'S GUIDE TO THE DASH DIET

50 DETAILED RECIPES TO INCREASE YOUR HEALTH AND PRODUCTIVITY TODAY

Table of Contents

Introduction

Potassium helps to lower the effects of sodium, which again, helps to lower down blood pressure, and that allows your body to experience a plethora of health benefits.

While the DASH diet primarily focuses on increasing the intake of fruits, vegetables, and low-fat dairy items, you are still allowed to go for meat-based recipes, although in small quantities.

For five years in a row, the DASH diet has been named the healthiest diet around by nutrition experts across the country. Originally designed to help lower blood pressure, it works almost as well as expensive prescription medications. The DASH diet (Dietary Approaches to Stop Hypertension) has also been shown to be instrumental in decreasing the risk of heart disease, stroke, cancer, and diabetes. It can lower your cholesterol, help prevent osteoporosis, and promote weight loss.

How can one diet plan do all that? The DASH diet is focused on increasing your intake of 'good carbs' such as fruits, vegetables, and whole grains. These replace the less healthy elements in your diet. In addition, the amount of sodium (salt) you consume is greatly decreased, replaced with healthier options for adding flavor and zest to your meals. Because processed foods are notoriously laden with salt, the DASH diet encourages the use of 'real' foods, foods fresh from your local market or frozen without additives.

Unlike many other popular diets, the DASH diet is easy to follow, very budget-friendly, and chock-full of variety. There are no 'forbidden' foods, no strange or unusual ingredients. Are you afraid that using unprocessed food will require hours in the kitchen? No way! Your trusty slow cooker (crock pot) can make it very easy to start eating healthier DASH diet meals immediately. Slow cooking imparts tremendous flavor to dishes by allowing the various ingredients enough time to blend their distinctive flavors. It's also easy on your finances since you can use less expensive cuts of meat and still have tender, succulent meals. In addition, your crockpot uses far less electricity, even running for 10 hours, than your stove or oven does. Definitely a win-win-win: health, flavor, budget! This book will explain why you need to adapt your eating habits, as well as how to implement that change. The recipes in this book are easy to prepare in your slow cooker, they'll give you DASH diet-friendly dishes to take you from appetizers and snacks through desserts … and they'll cook themselves while you get on with your life!

Are you ready to make a few simple changes that will improve your long-term health and help you to shed some excess baggage? Then dust off your crockpot, head to your kitchen, and read on!

Once you have decided your calorie intake, start your DASH diet by making incremental and gradual changes.

- An excellent way to start is to limit your sodium to 2,400 mg per day and reduce it eventually

- Once your body has adjusted itself to the change, go for 1,500 mg per day (which is about 2/3 spoon)

- (Keep in mind that the sodium count includes both the sodium already present in your food as well as any additional salt that you might add.) So, to summarize -

- Consume more fruits, low-fat dairy foods, and vegetables

- Try to cut back on foods that are high in cholesterol, saturated fat and trans fat

- Eat whole-grain foods, nuts, poultry and fish

- Try to limit sodium, sugary drinks, sweets and red meat, such as beef/pork, etc.

And you should be good to go!

How does the DASH diet promote weight loss and exercise? Despite not being specifically designed for weight loss, the Dash Diet does indeed help to trim down your weight through various indirect means.

While the DASH diet does not stress reductions in calories, it does influence you to fill up your diet with very nutrient-dense food as opposed to calorie-rich food, and this easily helps to shed a few pounds!

Since you will be on a heavy diet of veggies and fruits, you will be consuming lots of fiber, which is also believed to help in weight loss.

Aside from that, the diet also helps to control your appetite since cleaner and nutrient-dense foods will keep you satisfied throughout the day! Lower food intake will further contribute to weight loss.

And while you are at it, the program will indirectly encourage you to carry out a daily workout to keep your body healthy and fit. Following the DASH Diet program while working out will significantly enhance the effectiveness of the program.

Recipes

Breakfast

1 Heart-Friendly Sweet Potato-Oats Waffles

Preparation Time: 5 minutes

Cooking Time: 10 minutes

Servings: 2

Ingredients

For the waffles:

1 cup rolled oats

½ cup Sweet potato, cooked and skin removed

1 whole egg

1 egg white

1 cup almond milk

1 tablespoon honey

1 tablespoon olive oil

¼ teaspoon baking powder

¼ teaspoon salt

To serve:

Banana, sliced

Maple syrup

Directions

Preheat the waffle iron.

Meanwhile, add all the ingredients to a blender and process until pureed. Let the mixture stand for 10 minutes.

Coat the waffle iron with a nonstick cooking spray.

Pour ⅓ cup of the batter in each mold. Cook about 3-4 minutes per batch or 30 seconds longer after the light indicator turns green. Usually, waffles are done after the steam stops coming out of the waffle iron.

Serve with banana slices and maple syrup on top.

Nutrition:

Calories: 287

Carbohydrates: 54g

Fat: 8.39g

Saturated Fat: 1.6g

Fiber: 7.2g

Protein: 12.42g

Sodium: 285mg

Sugar: 22g

2 Whole-Grain Flax Waffles with Strawberry Purée

Preparation Time: 15 minutes

Cooking Time: 15 minutes

Serving: 6

Ingredients:

1-quart strawberries, hulled and chopped

1 cup water

2 tablespoons honey

2½ teaspoons pure vanilla extract, divided

2¼ cups whole-wheat flour

¼ cup ground flaxseed

2½ teaspoons baking powder

1 teaspoon baking soda

½ teaspoon kosher or sea salt

2 teaspoons ground cinnamon

2 tablespoons dark brown sugar

¼ cup canola oil

3 large eggs

1 cup nonfat milk

Cooking spray

Direction

First, make the strawberry purée: Place the strawberries, water, and honey and ½ teaspoon of vanilla extract in a medium saucepan. Bring to a simmer for 5 to 6 minutes, until the strawberries are soft. Use an immersion blender to purée the strawberries or transfer mixture to a blender and purée until smooth.

To make the waffles: In a medium mixing bowl, whisk together the flour, flaxseed, baking powder, baking soda, and salt until combined.

Scourge ground cinnamon, brown sugar, and canola oil until well combined. Whisk in one egg at a time until the mixture is fluffy. Add the remaining vanilla extract and milk until combined. Slowly whisk the dry ingredients into the wet mixture.

Heat a Belgian waffle maker over medium heat. Once hot, coat with the cooking spray. Evenly spoon 2/3 cup batter into the waffle maker. Shut the lid and cook for 1½ to 2 minutes, until the waffle is browned on the outside. Repeat with the remaining batter.

Serve the waffles with the strawberry purée.

Nutrition: 381 Calories 15g Total Fat 459mg Sodium 452mg Potassium 12g Protein

3 Blueberry Waffles

Preparation Time: 5 minutes

Cooking Time: 15 minutes

Serving: 8

Ingredients:

2 cups whole wheat flour

1 tablespoon baking powder

1 teaspoon ground cinnamon

2 tablespoons sugar

2 large eggs

3 tablespoons unsalted butter, melted

3 tablespoons nonfat plain Greek yogurt

1½ cups 1% milk

2 teaspoons vanilla extract

4 ounces blueberries

Nonstick cooking spray

½ cup maple almond butter

Direction

Preheat a waffle iron.

Mix flour, baking powder, cinnamon, and sugar.

Scourge eggs, melted butter, yogurt, milk, and vanilla.

Combine well.

Pour in wet ingredients to the dry mix and whisk until well combined. Do not over whisk; it's okay if the mixture has some lumps. Fold in the blueberries.

Coat the waffle iron with cooking spray. Scoop 1/3 cup of the batter onto the iron and cook until the waffles are lightly browned and slightly crisp. Repeat with the rest of the batter. Place 2 waffles in each of 4 storage containers. Store the almond butter in 4 condiment cups. To serve, top each warm waffle with 1 tablespoon of maple almond butter.

Nutrition: 647 Calories 37g Total fat 67g Carbohydrates 22g Protein 296mg Potassium 156mg Sodium

4 Apple Pancakes

Preparation Time: 5 minutes

Cooking Time: 9 minutes

Serving: 8

Ingredients:

¼ cup extra-virgin olive oil, divided

1 cup whole wheat flour

2 teaspoons baking powder

1 teaspoon baking soda

1 teaspoon ground cinnamon

1 cup 1% milk

2 large eggs

1 medium Gala apple, diced

2 tablespoons maple syrup

¼ cup chopped walnuts

Direction

Set aside 1 teaspoon of oil to use for oiling a griddle or skillet.

Mix the flour, baking powder, baking soda, cinnamon, milk, eggs, apple, and the remaining oil.

Heat a griddle or skillet over medium-high heat and coat with the reserved oil. Working in batches, pour in about ¼ cup of the batter for each pancake. Cook until browned on both sides.

Place 4 pancakes into each of 4 medium storage containers and the maple syrup in 4 small containers. To serve, drizzle each serving with 1 tablespoon of walnuts and drizzle with ½ tablespoon of maple syrup.

Nutrition: 378 Calories 22g Total fat 39g Carbohydrates 10g Protein 334mg Potassium 65mg Sodium

5 Peaches Mix

Preparation time: 10 minutes

Cooking time: 5 minutes

Servings: 4

Ingredients:

6 small peaches, cored and cut into wedges

¼ cup coconut sugar

2 tablespoons non-fat butter

¼ teaspoon almond extract

Directions:

In a small pan, combine the peaches with sugar, butter and almond extract, toss, cook over medium-high heat for 5 minutes, divide into bowls and serve for breakfast.

Enjoy!

Nutrition: calories 198, fat 2, fiber 6, carbs 11, protein 8

6 Cinnamon Brown Rice Pudding

Preparation time: 10 minutes

Cooking time: 25 minutes

Servings: 4

Ingredients:

1 cup brown rice

1 and ½ cups water

1 tablespoon vanilla extract

1 tablespoon cinnamon powder

1 tablespoon non-fat butter

½ cup coconut cream, unsweetened

Directions:

In a pot, combine the rice with the water, vanilla, cinnamon, butter and cream, stir, bring to a simmer over medium heat, cook for 25 minutes, divide into bowls and serve for breakfast.

Enjoy!

Nutrition: calories 182, fat 4, fiber 7, carbs 11, protein 6

7 Cream Basmati Rice Pudding

Preparation time: 10 minutes

Cooking time: 25 minutes

Servings: 6

Ingredients:

2 cups coconut milk

1 and ¼ cups water

1 cup basmati rice

2 tablespoons coconut sugar

¾ cup coconut cream

1 teaspoon vanilla extract

Directions:

In a pot, combine the coconut milk with the water, rice, sugar, cream and vanilla, toss, bring to a simmer over medium heat, cook for 25 minutes, stirring often, divide into bowls and serve for breakfast.

Enjoy!

Nutrition: calories 191, fat 4, fiber 7, carbs 11, protein 6

Soup

8 Roasted Carrot Soup

Preparation time: 15 minutes

Cooking time: 50 minutes

Servings: 4

Ingredients:

8 large carrots, washed and peeled

6 tablespoons olive oil

1-quart broth

Cayenne pepper to taste

Sunflower seeds and pepper to taste

Directions:

Warm your oven to 425 degrees F. Take a baking sheet, add carrots, drizzle olive oil, and roast for 30-45 minutes. Put roasted carrots into a blender and add broth, puree. Pour into saucepan and heat soup. Season with sunflower seeds, pepper and cayenne. Drizzle olive oil. Serve and enjoy!

Nutrition: Calories: 222 Fat: 18g Net Carbohydrates: 7g

Protein: 5g Sodium: 266 mg

9 Pumpkin Soup

Preparation time: 15 minutes

Cooking time: 6 hours

Servings: 4

Ingredients:

1 small pumpkin, halved, peeled, seeds removed, cubed

2 cups chicken broth

1 cup of coconut milk

Pepper and thyme to taste

Directions:

Add all the ingredients to a crockpot. Cook for 6-8 hours on low. Make a smooth puree by using a blender. Garnish with roasted seeds. Serve and enjoy!

Nutrition: Calories: 60 Fat: 2g Carbohydrates: 10g Protein: 3g Sodium: 10 mg

10   Coconut Avocado Soup

Preparation time: 15 minutes

Cooking time: 10 minutes

Servings: 4

Ingredients:

2 cups vegetable stock

2 teaspoons Thai green curry paste

Pepper as needed

1 avocado, chopped

1 tablespoon cilantro, chopped

Lime wedges

1 cup of coconut milk

Directions:

Add milk, avocado, curry paste, pepper to a blender, and blend. Take a pan and place it over medium heat. Add mixture and heat, simmer for 5 minutes. Stir in seasoning, cilantro, and simmer for 1 minute. Serve and enjoy!

Nutrition: Calories: 250 Fat: 30g Carbohydrates: 2g Protein: 4g Sodium: 378 mg

11   Coconut Arugula Soup

Preparation time: 15 minutes

Cooking time: 10 minutes

Servings: 4

Ingredients:

Black pepper as needed

1 tablespoon olive oil

2 tablespoons chives, chopped

2 garlic cloves, minced

10 ounces baby arugula

2 tablespoons tarragon, chopped

4 tablespoons coconut milk yogurt

6 cups chicken stock

2 tablespoons mint, chopped

1 onion, chopped

½ cup of coconut milk

Directions:

Take a saucepan and place it over medium-high heat, add oil and let it heat up. Put onion and garlic and fry within 5 minutes. Stir in stock and reduce the heat, let it simmer. Stir in tarragon, arugula, mint, parsley, and cook for 6 minutes. Mix in seasoning, chives, coconut yogurt, and serve. Nutrition: Calories: 180 Fat: 14g Carbohydrates: 20g Protein: 2g Sodium: 362 mg

12   Cabbage Soup

Preparation time: 15 minutes

Cooking time: 25 minutes

Servings: 3

Ingredients:

3 cups non-fat beef stock

2 garlic cloves, minced

1 tablespoon tomato paste

2 cups cabbage, chopped

½ yellow onion

½ cup carrot, chopped

½ cup green beans

½ cup zucchini, chopped

½ teaspoon basil

½ teaspoon oregano

Sunflower seeds and pepper as needed

Directions:

Grease a pot with non-stick cooking spray. Place it over medium heat and allow the oil to heat up. Add onions, carrots, and garlic, and sauté for 5 minutes. Add broth, tomato paste, green beans, cabbage, basil, oregano, sunflower seeds, and pepper.

Boil the whole mix and reduce the heat, simmer for 5-10 minutes until all veggies are tender. Add zucchini and simmer for 5 minutes more. Sever hot and enjoy!

Nutrition: Calories: 22 Fat: 0g Carbohydrates: 5g Protein: 1g Sodium: 200 mg

Meat

13   Easy Veal Chops

Preparation time: 10 minutes

Cooking time: 20 minutes

Servings: 4

Ingredients:

3 tablespoons whole wheat flour

Black pepper to the taste

2 eggs

1 tablespoon milk

1 and ½ cups whole wheat breadcrumbs

Zest of 1 lemon, grated

4 veal rib chops

3 tablespoons olive oil

Directions:

Put whole wheat flour in a bowl.

In another bowl, mix eggs with milk and whisk

In a third bowl, mix the breadcrumbs with lemon zest.

Season veal chops with black pepper, dredge them in flour, dip in the egg mix and then in breadcrumbs.

Heat up a pan with the oil over medium-high heat, add veal chops, cook for 2 minutes on each side and transfer to a baking sheet, introduce them in the oven at 350 degrees F, bake for 15 minutes, divide between plates and serve with a side salad.

Enjoy!

Nutrition: calories 270, fat 6, fiber 7, carbs 10, protein 16

14   Pork with Apple Sauce

Preparation time: 10 minutes

Cooking time: 1 hour and 30 minutes

Servings: 6

Ingredients:

1 tablespoon lemon juice

2 cups low-sodium veggie stock

17 ounces apples, cored and cut into wedges

2 pounds pork belly, trimmed and scored

1 teaspoons sweet paprika

Black pepper to the taste

A drizzle of olive oil

Directions:

In your blender, mix the stock with apples and lemon juice and pulse very well.

Put pork belly in a roasting pan, add apple sauce, also add the oil, paprika and black pepper, toss well, introduce in the oven and bake at 380 degrees F for 1 hour and 30 minutes.

Slice the pork belly, divide it between plates, drizzle the sauce all over and serve.

Enjoy!

Nutrition: calories 356, fat 14, fiber 4, carbs 10, protein 27

15   Citrus Pork

Preparation time: 10 minutes

Cooking time: 30 minutes

Servings: 4

Ingredients:

Zest of 2 limes, grated

Zest of 1 orange, grated

Juice of 1 orange

Juice of 2 limes

4 teaspoons garlic, minced

¾ cup olive oil

1 cup cilantro, chopped

1 cup mint, chopped

Black pepper to the taste

4 pork loin steaks

Directions:

In your food processor, mix lime zest and juice with orange zest and juice, garlic, oil, cilantro, mint and pepper and blend well.

Put the steaks in a bowl, add the citrus mix and toss really well.

Heat up a pan over medium-high heat, add pork steaks and the marinade, cook for 4 minutes on each side, introduce the pan in the oven and bake at 350 degrees F for 20 minutes.

Divide the steaks between plates, drizzle some of the cooking juices all over and serve with a side salad.

Enjoy!

Nutrition: calories 270, fat 7, fiber 2, carbs 8, protein 20

16   Pork Chops with Nutmeg

Preparation time: 10 minutes

Cooking time: 40 minutes

Servings: 3

Ingredients:

8 ounces mushrooms, sliced

¼ cup coconut milk

1 teaspoon garlic powder

1 yellow onion, chopped

3 pork chops, boneless

2 teaspoons nutmeg, ground

1 tablespoon balsamic vinegar

½ cup olive oil

Directions:

Heat up a pan with the oil over medium heat, add mushrooms and onions, stir and cook for 5 minutes.

Add pork chops, nutmeg and garlic powder and cook for 5 minutes more.

Add vinegar and coconut milk, toss, introduce in the oven and bake at 350 degrees F and bake for 30 minutes.

Divide between plates and serve.

Enjoy!

Nutrition: calories 260, fat 10, fiber 6, carbs 8, protein 22

17   Italian Parmesan Pork

Preparation time: 10 minutes

Cooking time: 30 minutes

Servings: 6

Ingredients:

2 tablespoons parsley, chopped

1 pound pork cutlets, thinly sliced

1 tablespoon olive oil

¼ cup yellow onion, chopped

3 garlic cloves, minced

2 tablespoons parmesan, grated

15 ounces canned tomatoes, no-salt-added and chopped

1/3 cup low sodium chicken stock

Black pepper to the taste

1 teaspoon Italian seasoning

Directions:

Heat up a pan with the oil over medium-high heat, add pork cutlets, season with Italian seasoning and black pepper and cook for 4 minutes on each side.

Add onion, garlic, tomatoes, stock and top with parmesan, introduce the pan in the oven and bake at 350 degrees F for 20 minutes.

Sprinkle parsley on top, divide everything between plates and serve.

Enjoy!

Nutrition: calories 280, fat 17, fiber 5, carbs 12, protein 34

18   Pork Roast with Cranberry

Preparation time: 10 minutes

Cooking time: 1 hour and 30 minutes

Servings: 4

Ingredients:

1 tablespoon coconut flour

Black pepper to the taste

1 and ½ pounds pork loin roast

½ teaspoon ginger, grated

½ cup cranberries

2 garlic cloves, minced

Juice of ½ lemon

½ cup low-sodium veggie stock

Directions:

Put the stock in a small pan, heat it up over medium-high heat, add black pepper, ginger, garlic, cranberries, lemon juice and the flour, whisk well and cook for 10 minutes.

Put the roast in a pan, add the cranberry sauce on top, introduce in the oven and bake at 375 degrees F for 1 hour and 20 minutes.

Slice the roast, divide it and the sauce between plates and serve.

Enjoy!

Nutrition: calories 330, fat 13, fiber 2, carbs 13, protein 25

Seafood

19   Shrimp and Orzo

Preparation time: 10 minutes

Cooking time: 30 minutes

Servings: 4

Ingredients:

1 pound shrimp, peeled and deveined

Black pepper to the taste

3 garlic cloves, minced

1 tablespoon olive oil

½ teaspoon oregano, dried

1 yellow onion, chopped

2 cups low-sodium chicken stock

2 ounces orzo

½ cup water

4 ounces canned tomatoes, no-salt-added and chopped

Juice of 1 lemon

Directions:

Heat up a pan with the oil over medium-high heat, add onion, garlic and oregano, stir and cook for 4 minutes.

Add orzo, stir and cook for 2 more minutes.

Add stock and the water, bring to a boil, cover, reduce heat to low and cook for 12 minutes.

Add lemon juice, tomatoes, black pepper and shrimp, introduce in the oven and bake at 400 degrees F for 15 minutes.

Divide between plates and serve.

Enjoy!

Nutrition: calories 228, fat 4, fiber 3, carbs 7, protein 8

20   Lemon and Garlic Scallops

Preparation time: 10 minutes

Cooking Time: 5 minutes

Serving: 4

Ingredients:

1 tablespoon olive oil

1 ¼ pounds dried scallops

2 tablespoons all-purpose flour

¼ teaspoon sunflower seeds

4-5 garlic cloves, minced

1 scallion, chopped

1 pinch of ground sage

1 lemon juice

2 tablespoons parsley, chopped

Direction

Take a nonstick skillet and place over medium-high heat.

Add oil and allow the oil to heat up.

Take a medium sized bowl and add scallops alongside sunflower seeds and flour.

Place the scallops in the skillet and add scallions, garlic, and sage.

Sauté for 3-4 minutes until they show an opaque texture.

Stir in lemon juice and parsley.

Remove heat and serve hot!

Nutrition:

Calories: 151

Fat: 4g

Carbohydrates: 10g

Protein: 18g

21   Walnut Encrusted Salmon

Preparation time: 10 minutes

Cooking Time: 14 minutes

Serving: 34

Ingredients:

½ cup walnuts

2 tablespoons stevia

½ tablespoon Dijon mustard

¼ teaspoon dill

2 salmon fillets (3 ounces each)

1 tablespoon olive oil

Sunflower seeds and pepper to taste

Directions:

Preheat your oven to 350 degrees F.

Add walnuts, mustard, stevia to food processor and process until your desired consistency is achieved.

Take a frying pan and place it over medium heat.

Add oil and let it heat up.

Add salmon and sear for 3 minutes.

Add walnut mix and coat well.

Transfer coated salmon to baking sheet, bake in oven for 8 minutes.

Serve and enjoy!

Nutrition:

Calories: 373

Fat: 43g

Carbohydrates: 4g

Protein: 20g

22 Roasted Lemon Swordfish

Preparation time: 10 minutes

Cooking Time: 70-80 minutes

Serving: 4

Ingredients:

¼ cup parsley, chopped

½ teaspoon garlic, chopped

½ teaspoon canola oil

4 swordfish fillets, 6 ounces each

¼ teaspoon sunflower seeds

1 tablespoon sugar

2 lemons, quartered and seeds removed

Directions:

Preheat your oven to 375 degrees F.

Take a small-sized bowl and add sugar, sunflower seeds, lemon wedges.

Toss well to coat them.

Take a shallow baking dish and add lemons, cover with aluminum foil.

Roast for about 60 minutes until lemons are tender and browned (Slightly).

Heat your grill and place the rack about 4 inches away from the source of heat.

Take a baking pan and coat it with cooking spray.

Transfer fish fillets to the pan and brush with oil on top spread garlic on top.

Grill for about 5 minutes each side until fillet turns opaque.

Transfer fish to a serving platter, squeeze roasted lemon on top.

Sprinkle parsley serve with a lemon wedge on the side.

Enjoy!

Nutrition:

Calories: 280

Fat: 12g

Net Carbohydrates: 4g

Protein: 34g

Vegetarian and Vegan

23   Carrot Cakes

Preparation Time: 10 minutes

Cooking Time: 10 minutes

Servings: 4

Ingredients:

1 cup carrot, grated

1 tablespoon semolina

1 egg, beaten

1 teaspoon Italian seasonings

1 tablespoon sesame oil

Directions:

In the mixing bowl, mix up grated carrot, semolina, egg, and Italian seasonings.

Heat up sesame oil in the skillet.

Make the carrot cakes with the help of 2 spoons and put in the skillet.

Roast the cakes for 4 minutes per side.

Nutrition:

Calories 70

Protein 1.9g

Carbohydrates 4.8g

Fat 4.9g

Fiber 0.8g

Cholesterol 42mg

Sodium 35mg

Potassium 108mg

24   Vegan Chili

Preparation Time: 10 minutes

Cooking Time: 25 minutes

Servings: 4

Ingredients:

½ cup bulgur

1 cup tomatoes, chopped

1 chili pepper, chopped

1 cup red kidney beans, cooked

2 cups low-sodium chicken broth

1 teaspoon tomato paste

½ cup celery stalk, chopped

Directions:

Put all ingredients in the big saucepan and stir well.

Close the lid and simmer the chili for 25 minutes over the medium-low heat.

Nutrition:

Calories 234

Protein 14.1g

Carbohydrates 44.4g

Fat 0.9g

Fiber 1g

Cholesterol 0mg

Sodium 57mg

Potassium 52mg

25   Spinach Casserole

Preparation Time: 5 minutes

Cooking Time: 30 minutes

Servings: 3

Ingredients:

2 cups spinach, chopped

4 oz artichoke hearts, chopped

¼ cup low-fat yogurt

1 teaspoon Italian seasonings

2 oz vegan mozzarella, shredded

Directions:

Mix up all ingredients in the casserole mold and cover it with foil.

Then transfer it in the preheated to 365F oven and bake it for 30 minutes.

Nutrition:

Calories 102

Protein 3.7g

Carbohydrates 11g

Fat 4.9g

Fiber 2.5g

Cholesterol 2mg

Sodium 206mg

Potassium 300mg

26   Tofu Turkey

Preparation Time: 15 minutes

Cooking Time: 75 minutes

Servings: 6

Ingredients:

1 onion, diced

1 cup mushrooms, chopped

1 bell pepper, chopped

12 oz firm tofu, crumbled

1 teaspoon dried rosemary

1 tablespoon avocado oil

½ cup marinara sauce

1 teaspoon miso paste

Directions:

Sauté onion, mushrooms, bell pepper, rosemary, miso paste, and avocado oil in the saucepan until the ingredients are cooked (appx.10-15 minutes).

Then put ½ part of tofu in the round baking pan. Press well and make the medium whole in the center.

Put the mushroom mixture in the tofu whole and top it with marinara sauce.

Add remaining tofu and press it well. Cover the meal with foil.

Bake the tofu turkey for 60 minutes at 395F.

Nutrition:

Calories 80

Protein 5.9g

Carbohydrates 7.9g

Fat 3.4

Fiber 2.1g

Cholesterol 0mg

Sodium 130mg

Potassium 262mg

27   Cauliflower Tots

Preparation Time: 15 minutes

Cooking Time: 20 minutes

Servings: 4

Ingredients:

1 cup cauliflower, shredded

3 oz vegan Parmesan, grated

1/3 cup flax seeds meal

1 egg, beaten

1 teaspoon Italian seasonings

1 teaspoon olive oil

Directions:

In the bowl mix up shredded cauliflower, vegan Parmesan, flax seeds meal, egg, and Italian seasonings.

Knead the cauliflower mixture. Add water if needed.

After this, make the cauliflower tots from the mixture.

Line the baking tray with baking paper and place the cauliflower tots inside.

Sprinkle them with the olive oil and transfer in the preheated to 375F oven.

Bake the meal for 15-20 minutes or until golden brown.

Nutrition:

Calories 109

Protein 6.1g

Carbohydrates 6.3g

Fat 6.6g

Fiber 3.7g

Cholesterol 42mg

Sodium 72mg

Potassium 158mg

Side Dishes, Salads & Appetizers

28   Interesting Tofu Spinach

Preparation time: 5 minutes

Cooking time: 18 minutes

Servings: 2

Ingredients:

10 ounces of washed Spinach

1 ounce of firm Tofu

1 chopped up onion

1 chopped up tomato

2 pieces of Red Whole Chili

5 cloves of Garlic

1-inch piece of Ginger

1 tablespoon of oil

Coconut for garnish

Spices

1 teaspoon of cumin seeds

1 teaspoon of coriander

½ a teaspoon of Cayenne powder

½ a teaspoon of Cayenne powder

¼ teaspoon of Garam masala

1 teaspoon of flavored vinegar

Directions:

Press your tofu and drain any excess water

Cut the tofu into small sized cubes

Add 2 tablespoon of oil to a saucepan and place it over medium heat

Add tofu and brown on all side for 5 minutes

Transfer the browned tofu to a plate and keep them on the side

Set your pot to Sauté mode and add 1 tablespoon of oil, cumin seeds

Toast the cumin and add garlic, onion, ginger, red chili and sauté for 3 minutes

Stir in spices and tomato

Add spinach and lock up the lid

Cook on HIGH pressure for 2 minutes

Once done, release the pressure naturally and blend the contents using an immersion blender

Set the pot to Sauté mode once more and add fried tofu, cook for 1 minute more

Garnish with a bit of coconut and enjoy!

Nutrition: 155 Calories 11g Fat 16g Carbohydrates 2g Protein 161mg Potassium 74mg Sodium

29   Mexican Crazy Polenta

Preparation time: 5 minutes

Cooking time: 15 minutes

Servings: 2

Ingredients:

1 cup of sliced green onion

2 teaspoons of minced garlic

2 cups of vegetable broth

2 cups of water

1 cup of corn meal grits

¼ cup of freshly chopped cilantro

1 teaspoon of cumin

1 teaspoon of oregano

1 /2 a teaspoon of smoked paprika

¼ teaspoon of cayenne pepper

Directions:

Set the pot to Sauté mode

Add minced garlic, onion and Sauté for 2-3 minutes

Add vegetable broth, water, spice, cilantro and corn meal

Mix

Close and cook at HIGH pressure for 5 minutes

Release the pressure naturally over 10 minutes

Stir and enjoy!

Nutrition: 731 Calories 26g Fat 10g Carbohydrates 20g Protein 201mg Potassium 69mg Sodium

30   Egg and Bean Medley

Preparation time: 5 minutes

Cooking time: 18 minutes

Servings: 2

Ingredients:

½ a cup of milk

5 beaten eggs

½ a cup of tomato sauce

1 cup of cooked up white beans

2 chopped up cloves of garlic

1 teaspoon of chili powder

Directions:

Pour milk and eggs to a bowl and mix well

Add the rest of the ingredients and mix well

Stir in 1 cup of water to the pot

Transfer the bowl to your pot and lock up the lid

Cook on HIGH pressure for 18 minutes

Release the pressure naturally over 10 minutes

Serve with warm bread

Enjoy!

Nutrition: 206 Calories 9g Fat 23g Carbohydrates 9g Protein 181 mg Potassium 70mg Sodium

31   Healthy Potatouille

Preparation time: 5 minutes

Cooking time: 10 minutes

Servings: 2

Ingredients:

½ a cup of water

8 ounces of yellow Crookneck Squash

8 ounces of Zucchini

12 ounces of Chinese Eggplant

1 piece of Orange bell pepper

2-3 Portobello mushroom

½ a red onion chopped up

24 ounce of Yukon gold potatoes

2 cans of fire roasted tomatoes

½ a cup of basil, fresh chopped up into threads

Directions:

Add the listed ingredients to your Instant Pot

Close and cook at HIGH pressure for 10 minutes

Once done, perform a quick release

Open the lid and stir in basil

Serve it over rice. Enjoy!

Nutrition: 731 Calories 26g Fat 16g Carbohydrates 20g Protein 111mg Potassium 73mg Sodium

32   Fancy Red and White Sprouts

Preparation time: 10 minutes

Cooking time: 3 minutes

Servings: 2

Ingredients:

1 pound of Brussels sprouts

¼ cup of pine nuts toasted

1 pomegranate

1 tablespoon of extra virgin olive oil

½ a teaspoon of flavored vinegar

1 grate pepper

Directions:

Pull out outer leaves and trim the stems

Wash the Brussels

Cut the largest one in half and get all the ones in uniform size

Add 1 cup of water. Put steamer basket

Add sprouts to steamer basket

close and cook at HIGH pressure for 3 minutes

Release the pressure naturally

Move sprouts to serving dish and dress with olive oil, pepper and flavored vinegar

Sprinkle toasted pine nuts and pomegranate seeds. Serve and enjoy!

Nutrition: 197 Calories 7g Fat 22g Carbohydrates 6g Protein 177mg Potassium 63mg Sodium

33   Garlic and Chive "Mash"

Preparation time: 8 minutes

Cooking time: 8 minutes

Servings: 2

Ingredients:

2 cups of vegetable stock

2 pound of peeled Yukon potatoes

4 cloves of peeled garlic

½ a cup of almond milk

½ a teaspoon of flavored vinegar

¼ cup of chives chopped up

Directions:

Add broth, garlic and potatoes to the Instant Pot

Lock up the lid and cook on HIGH pressure for 9 minutes

Release the pressure naturally over 10 minutes

Drain just the amount of liquid required to maintain your required consistency

Mash the potatoes and stir in flavored vinegar and milk

Stir in chives and serve

Enjoy!

Nutrition: 293 Calories 14g Fat 35g Carbohydrates 8g Protein 122mg Potassium 81mg Sodium

34   Garlic and Broccoli Mishmash

Preparation time: 3 minutes

Cooking time: 12 minutes

Servings: 2

Ingredients:

1-2 broccoli head cut up into florets

1`/2 a cup of water

6 cloves of minced garlic

1 tablespoon of peanut oil

White Wine Vinegar

Sea flavored vinegar

Directions:

Place a steamer rack in your cooker. Add the florets to the rack

Pour in ½ cup of water to the pot

Lock up the lid and cook on LOW pressure for 0 minutes. Quick release

Allow the broccoli to cool by transferring them to an ice bath

Remove water and set the pot to Sauté mode

Add 1 tablespoon of peanut oil alongside minced garlic

Sauté for 25-30 seconds and add the broccoli alongside 1 tablespoon of white wine vinegar

Season with a bit of flavored vinegar and stir for 30 seconds.

Enjoy!

Nutrition: 101 Calories 8g Fat 6g Carbohydrates 6g Protein 131mg Potassium 74mg Sodium

35   Crashing Asparagus Risotto with Micro stock

Preparation time: 10 minutes

Cooking time: 10 minutes

Servings: 2

Ingredients:

1 pound of asparagus

4 cups of water

2 tablespoon of olive oil

1 medium size chopped red oni0on

2 cups of Arborio rice

¼ cup of white wine vinegar

2 teaspoons of flavored vinegar

½ a teaspoon of lemon juice

Directions:

Cut asparagus by removing the stem, wash them under cold water and slice them in rondels making sure to keep the tips

Add woody stems and water to your Instant Pot

Seal and cook at HIGH pressure for 12 minutes, release the pressure naturally

Lift up the woody stem and pour out the cooking liquid

Pour the liquid into a measuring cup

Add onion, olive oil to the pot and swirl

Add rice, onion and stir

Cook for 2 minutes

Drizzle a bit of wine vinegar and deglaze

Add asparagus micro stock, asparagus rondels and tips

Season with flavored vinegar

Lock up the lid and cook on HIGH pressure for 6 minutes

Release the pressure naturally

Add a squeeze of lemon juice and serve

Enjoy!

Nutrition: 486 Calories 7g Fat 71g Carbohydrates 37g Protein 142mg Potassium 88mg Sodium

36   Crunchy Creamy Mashed Sweet Potatoes

Preparation time: 5 minutes

Cooking time: 20 minutes

Servings: 2

Ingredients:

2 pound of garnet sweet potatoes cut up into 1-inch chunks

2-3 tablespoon of vegan butter

2 tablespoon of maple syrup

¼ teaspoon of nutmeg

1 cup of water

Sea flavored vinegar as needed

Directions:

Peel the sweet potatoes and cut up into 1-inch chunks

Pour 1 cup of water to the pot and add steamer basket. Add sweet potato chunks in the basket

Lock up the lid and cook on HIGH pressure for 8 minutes

Quick release the pressure

Open the lid and place the cooked sweet potatoes to the bowl

Use a masher to mash the potatoes

Add ¼ teaspoon of nutmeg, 2-3 tablespoon of unflavored vinegar butter, 2 tablespoon of maple syrup. Mash and mix

Season with flavored vinegar. Serve and enjoy!

Nutrition: 249 Calories 8g Fat 37g Carbohydrates 7g Protein 133mg Potassium 69mg Sodium

37   Tasty Yogurt and Cucumber Salad

Serving: 4

Preparation time: 10 minutes

Cooking Time: Nil

Ingredients:

5-6 small cucumbers, peeled and diced

1 (8 ounces) container plain Greek yogurt

2 garlic cloves, minced

1 tablespoon fresh mint, minced

Sea sunflower seeds and fresh black pepper

Directions:

Take a large bowl and add cucumbers, garlic, yogurt, mint.

Season with sunflower seeds and pepper.

Refrigerate the salad for 1 hour and serve.

Enjoy!

Nutrition:

Calories: 74

Fat: 0.7g

Carbohydrates: 16g

Protein: 2g

Dessert and Snacks

38   Sensational Strawberry Medley

Preparation time: 5 minutes

Serving: 2

Ingredients:

1-2 handful baby greens

3 medium kale leaves

5-8 mint leaves

1 inch piece ginger , peeled

1 avocado

1 cup strawberries

6-8 ounces coconut water + 6-8 ounces filtered water

Fresh juice of one lime

1-2 teaspoon olive oil

Directions:

Add all the listed ingredients to your blender.

Blend until smooth.

Add a few ice cubes and serve the smoothie.

Enjoy!

Nutrition:

Calories: 200

Fat: 10g

Carbohydrates: 14g

Protein 2g

39   Sweet Almond and Coconut Fat Bombs

Preparation time: 10 minutes

Serving: 6

Cooking Time: /Freeze Time: 20 minutes

Ingredients:

¼ cup melted coconut oil

9 ½ tablespoons almond butter

90 drops liquid stevia

3 tablespoons cocoa

9 tablespoons melted butter, salted

Directions:

Take a bowl and add all of the listed ingredients.

Mix them well.

Pour scant 2 tablespoons of the mixture into as many muffin molds as you like.

Chill for 20 minutes and pop them out.

Serve and enjoy!

Nutrition:

Total Carbs: 2g

Fiber: 0g

Protein: 2.53g

Fat: 14g

40   Almond and Tomato Balls

Preparation time: 10 minutes

Cooking Time: /Freeze Time: 20 minutes

Serving: 6

Ingredients:

1/3 cup pistachios, de-shelled

10 ounces cream cheese

1/3 cup sun dried tomatoes, diced

Directions:

Chop pistachios into small pieces.

Add cream cheese, tomatoes in a bowl and mix well.

Chill for 15-20 minutes and turn into balls.

Roll into pistachios.

Serve and enjoy!

Nutrition:

Carb: 183

Fat: 18g

Carb: 5g

Protein: 5g

41   Avocado Tuna Bites

Preparation time: 10 minutes

Cooking Time: Nil

Serving: 4

Ingredients:

1/3 cup coconut oil

1 avocado, cut into cubes

10 ounces canned tuna, drained

¼ cup parmesan cheese, grated

¼ teaspoon garlic powder

1/4 teaspoon onion powder

1/3 cup almond flour

¼ teaspoon pepper

¼ cup low fat mayonnaise

Pepper as needed

Directions:

Take a bowl and add tuna, mayo, flour, parmesan, spices and mix well.

Fold in avocado and make 12 balls out of the mixture.

Melt coconut oil in pan and cook over medium heat, until all sides are golden.

Serve and enjoy!

Nutrition:

Calories: 185

Fat: 18g

Carbohydrates: 1g

Protein: 5g

42 Mediterranean Pop Corn Bites

Preparation time: 5 minutes + 20 minutes chill time

Cooking Time: 2-3 minutes

Serving: 4

Ingredients:

3 cups Medjool dates, chopped

12 ounces brewed coffee

1 cup pecan, chopped

½ cup coconut, shredded

½ cup cocoa powder

Directions:

Soak dates in warm coffee for 5 minutes.

Remove dates from coffee and mash them, making a fine smooth mixture.

Stir in remaining ingredients (except cocoa powder) and form small balls out of the mixture.

Coat with cocoa powder, serve and enjoy!

Nutrition:

Calories: 265

Fat: 12g

Carbohydrates: 43g

Protein 3g

43   Hearty Buttery Walnuts

Preparation time: 10 minutes

Cooking Time: Nil

Serving: 4

Ingredients:

4 walnut halves

½ tablespoon almond butter

Directions:

Spread butter over two walnut halves.

Top with other halves.

Serve and enjoy!

Nutrition:

Calories: 90

Fat: 10g

Carbohydrates: 0g

Protein: 1g

Preparation time: 20 minutes + 20 hours chill time

Cooking Time: Nil

Serving: 4

Ingredients:

4 cups watermelon, seedless and chunked

¼ cup coconut sugar

2 tablespoons lime juice

Directions:

Add the listed ingredients to a blender and puree.

Transfer to a freezer container with a tight-fitting lid.

Freeze the mix for about 4-6 hours until you have gelatin-like consistency.

Puree the mix once again in batches and return to the container.

Chill overnight.

Allow the sorbet to stand for 5 minutes before serving and enjoy!

Nutrition:

Calories: 91

Fat: 0g

Carbohydrates: 25g

Protein: 1g

45   Lovely Faux Mac and Cheese

Preparation time: 15 minutes

Cooking Time: 45 minutes

Serving: 4

Ingredients:

5 cups cauliflower florets

Salt and pepper to taste

1 cup coconut milk

½ cup vegetable broth

2 tablespoons coconut flour, sifted

1 organic egg, beaten

2 cups cheddar cheese

Directions:

Preheat your oven to 350 degrees F.

Season florets with salt and steam until firm.

Place florets in greased ovenproof dish.

Heat coconut milk over medium heat in a skillet, make sure to season the oil with salt and pepper.

Stir in broth and add coconut flour to the mix, stir.

Cook until the sauce begins to bubble.

Remove heat and add beaten egg.

Pour the thick sauce over cauliflower and mix in cheese.

Bake for 30-45 minutes.

Serve and enjoy!

Nutrition:

Calories: 229

Fat: 14g

Carbohydrates: 9g

Protein: 15g

46   Beautiful Banana Custard

Preparation time: 10 minutes

Cooking Time: 25 minutes

Serving: 3

Ingredients:

2 ripe bananas, peeled and mashed finely

½ teaspoon of vanilla extract

14-ounce unsweetened almond milk

3 eggs

Directions:

Preheat your oven to 350 degrees F.

Grease 8 custard glasses lightly.

Arrange the glasses in a large baking dish.

Take a large bowl and mix all of the ingredients and mix them well until combined nicely.

Divide the mixture evenly between the glasses.

Pour water in the baking dish.

Bake for 25 minutes.

Take out and serve.

Enjoy!

Nutrition:

Calories: 59

Fat: 2.4g

Carbohydrates: 7g

Protein: 3g

47   Healthy Tahini Buns

Preparation time: 10 minutes

Cooking Time: 15-20 minutes

Serving: 3 buns Ingredients:

1 whole egg

5 tablespoons Tahini paste

½ teaspoon baking soda

1 teaspoon lemon juice

1 pinch salt

Directions:

Preheat your oven to 350 degrees F.

Line a baking sheet with parchment paper and keep it on the side.

Add the listed ingredients to a blender and blend until you have a smooth batter.

Scoop batter onto prepared sheet forming buns.

Bake for 15-20 minutes.

Once done, remove from oven and let them cool.

Serve and enjoy!

Nutrition:

Total Carbs: 7g

Fiber: 2g

Protein: 6g

Fat: 14g

Calories: 172

48   Spicy Pecan Bowl

Preparation time: 10 minutes

Cooking Time: 120 minutes

Serving: 3

Ingredients:

1 pound pecans, halved

2 tablespoons olive oil

1 teaspoon basil, dried

1 tablespoon chili powder

1 teaspoon oregano, dried

¼ teaspoon garlic powder

1 teaspoon rosemary, dried

½ teaspoon onion powder

Directions:

Add pecans, oil, basil, chili powder, oregano, garlic powder, onion powder, rosemary and toss well.

Transfer to Slow Cooker and cook on LOW for 2 hours.

Divide between bowls and serve.

Enjoy!

Nutrition:

Calories: 152

Fat: 3g

Carbohydrates: 11g

Protein: 2g

49   Gentle Sweet Potato Tempura

Preparation time: 15 minutes

Cooking Time: 4 minutes

Serving: 4

Ingredients:

2 whole eggs

½ teaspoon salt

3/4 cup ice water + 3 tablespoons ice water

¾ cup all-purpose flour + 1 tablespoons all-purpose flour

2 cups oil

1 sweet potato, scrubbed and sliced into 1/8 inch slices

For sauce

¼ cup rice wine

¼ cup coconut aminos

Directions:

Take a large bowl and beat in eggs until frothy.

Stir in salt, ice water, and flour, mix well until the batter is lumpy.

Take a frying pan and place over high heat, add oil and heat to 350 degrees F.

Dry-sweet potato slices and dip 3 slices at a time in the batter, let excess batter drip.

Fry until golden brown on both sides, each side should take about 2 minutes.

Live them out and drain excess oil, keep repeating until all potatoes are done.

Take a small bowl and whisk in rice wine, soy sauce and use it as a dipping sauce.

Enjoy!

Nutrition:

Calories: 315

Fat: 13g

Carbohydrates: 35g

Protein: 8g

50   Terrific Jalapeno Bacon Bombs

Preparation time: 15 minutes

Cooking time: 10 minutes

Servings: 2

Ingredients:

12 large jalapeno peppers

16 bacon strips

6 ounces full fat cream cheese

2 teaspoon garlic powder

1 teaspoon chili powder

Directions:

Preheat your oven to 350 degrees F.

Place a wire rack over a roasting pan and keep it on the side.

Make a slit lengthways across jalapeno pepper and scrape out the seeds, discard them.

Place a nonstick skillet over high heat and add half of your bacon strips, cook until crispy.

Drain them.

Chop the cooked bacon strips and transfer to large bowl.

Add cream cheese and mix.

Season the cream cheese and bacon mix with garlic and chili powder.

Mix well.

Stuff the mix into the jalapeno peppers with and wrap a raw bacon strip all around.

Arrange the stuffed wrapped jalapeno on prepared wire rack.

Roast for 10 minutes.

Transfer to cooling rack and serve!

Nutrition: Calories: 209 Fat: 9g Net Carbohydrates: 15g Protein: 9g

Conclusion

Thank you for taking the time to read this book on the DASH diet! We sincerely hope that the book was educational and helpful.

We also hope that you will take the lessons of the DASH diet to heart. Namely that you can take charge of your own health.

Remember what grandma said – you are what you eat.

And it's true!

If you found this book useful and informative, please drop by and give us a review!

Thanks for reading, and good luck with your health!

CPSIA information can be obtained
at www.ICGtesting.com
Printed in the USA
BVHW041408050321
601819BV00007B/217